Acid Reflux Cookbook for Beginners

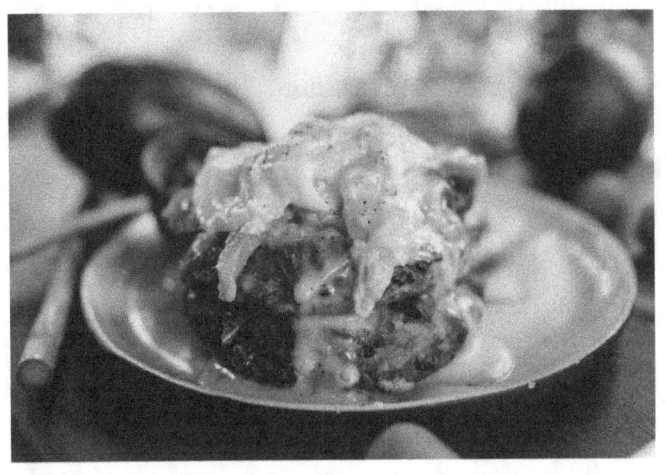

100 Days of Delicious and Nourishing Recipes and 8-weeks Meal Plan to Combat, GERD & LPR Symptoms, Overcome Discomfort and Achieve Well-being

Dr. Teresa J. West

TABLE OF CONTENTS

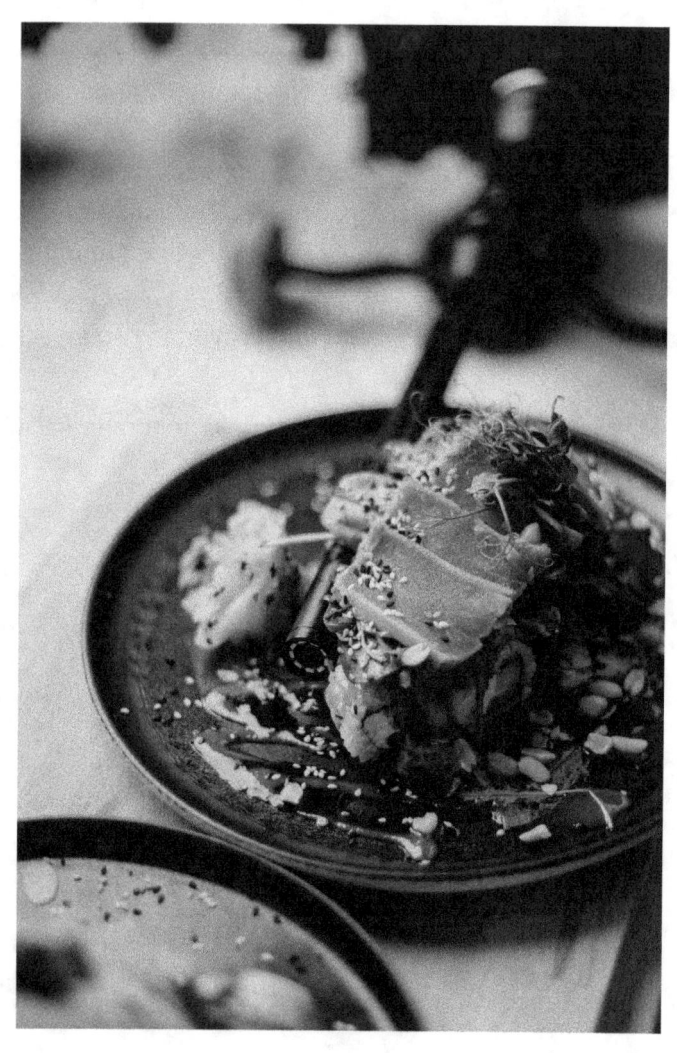

Introduction

Suffering from acid reflux is a widespread issue affecting millions globally, manifesting as the regurgitation of stomach acid into the esophagus, resulting in the discomforting sensation commonly known as heartburn. This condition not only brings about an uneasy feeling but can also lead to complications such as difficulty swallowing, persistent coughing, and even dental problems due to prolonged exposure to stomach acid.

For those grappling with acid reflux, finding effective relief can be a daunting task. While medications can provide some assistance, an increasing number of individuals are turning to lifestyle and dietary adjustments to manage their symptoms more holistically. This is where the significance of this acid reflux cookbook tailored for beginners comes into play.

This acid reflux cookbook designed for beginners serves as a valuable resource to aid individuals in making informed food choices that alleviate discomfort and enhance overall well-being. It features a diverse array of delectable, easy-to-prepare recipes crafted to be gentle on the digestive system, minimizing the likelihood of triggering acid reflux symptoms.

Within the pages of this cookbook, one can anticipate discovering recipes that are not only low in fat and acidity but also rich in fiber and essential nutrients. Examples of these palate-pleasing dishes may include comforting options like banana-infused oatmeal, healthful choices such as grilled chicken with an assortment of vegetables, and even indulgent yet reflux-friendly desserts like apple crisp and banana bread. Beyond recipes, the cookbook may offer insights into meal planning and portion control, facilitating the creation of a well-balanced diet conducive to digestive health.

However, the utility of this acid reflux cookbook for beginners extends beyond its recipes. It often provides valuable information elucidating the causes and symptoms of acid reflux, coupled with practical guidance on effecting positive changes in eating habits. It even went the extra mile by incorporating comprehensive meal plans and convenient shopping lists, streamlining the process of transitioning towards a diet that supports digestive well-being.

Whether you're a novice in the kitchen or someone seeking effective ways to manage acid reflux, this beginner's cookbook proves to be an invaluable companion. It empowers individuals to assume control over their health and well-being through mindful food choices, presenting a novel and enjoyable approach to mitigating acid reflux symptoms.

Chapter 1

Understanding Acid Reflux

Acid reflux, medically termed gastroesophageal reflux disease (GERD), is a prevalent ailment affecting millions globally. This condition transpires when stomach acid regurgitates into the esophagus, giving rise to symptoms such as heartburn, chest pain, and difficulty swallowing. A comprehensive comprehension of the causes, symptoms, and triggers of acid reflux is imperative for effective management and an improved quality of life.

Within this chapter, we embark on an exploration of the fundamentals of acid reflux, delve into common symptoms and triggers, and scrutinize the profound impact of dietary choices on this condition. Moreover, we will investigate how adopting dietary modifications can mitigate symptoms and enhance overall health.

What is Acid Reflux?

Acid reflux unfolds when the lower esophageal sphincter (LES), a muscular ring situated at the esophagus's base, fails to close adequately. This malfunction permits stomach acid to surge back into the esophagus, sparking irritation and inflammation of the esophageal lining. Consequently, a spectrum of symptoms, including heartburn, regurgitation, and chest pain, emerges. While sporadic acid reflux episodes are considered normal, frequent occurrences may indicate the presence of GERD, a chronic and more severe manifestation of the condition.

Common Symptoms and Triggers

Manifestations of acid reflux exhibit variability from one individual to another; nonetheless, prevalent indicators encompass:

Some common symptoms include :

- Heartburn: a fiery sensation in the chest, often exacerbated after meals or when lying down.
- Regurgitation: the perception of acid flowing back into the throat or mouth.
- Chest pain: a sensation of pressure or discomfort in the chest, occasionally confused with a heart attack.
- Difficulty swallowing: the feeling of food sticking in the throat or chest.

In tandem with these symptoms, specific triggers can exacerbate acid reflux, including:

Some common triggers include :

- High-fat foods: the consumption of fried and oily foods can relax the LES, promoting acid reflux.
- Citrus fruits: oranges, lemons, and grapefruits, owing to their acidity, can irritate the esophagus.
- Spicy foods: the inclusion of hot peppers and spices can incite heartburn and chest pain.
- Alcohol and caffeine: these substances can induce LES relaxation and augment stomach acid production.

- **Smoking:** exposure to tobacco smoke can weaken the LES, contributing to acid reflux.

The Impact of Diet on Acid Reflux

Diet exerts a substantial influence on both the onset and management of acid reflux. Certain edibles and beverages can exacerbate symptoms, while others can provide relief and enhance overall digestive well-being. Incorporating dietary alterations is a pivotal aspect of acid reflux management, reducing the risk of complications such as esophagitis and Barrett's esophagus.

Foods to Avoid:

- **High-fat foods:** minimizing the intake of fried foods, full-fat dairy, and fatty meats can help prevent acid reflux.
- **Citrus fruits:** Stepping clear of acidic fruits like oranges and grapefruits can alleviate heartburn and regurgitation.

- Spicy foods: limiting the consumption of hot peppers, garlic, and onions can mitigate acid reflux, especially in large quantities.
- Chocolate: due to its methylxanthine content, chocolate can relax the LES, fostering acid reflux.
- Carbonated beverages: avoiding sodas and carbonated drinks is crucial, as they can induce bloating and heighten LES pressure, leading to acid reflux.

Foods to Incorporate:

- Lean proteins: opting for chicken, turkey, fish, and plant-based proteins facilitates easier digestion, lessening the likelihood of triggering acid reflux.
- Non-citrus fruits: including apples, bananas, and melons in the diet provides lower-acid alternatives that are gentler on the esophagus.
- Vegetables: integrating leafy greens, broccoli, cauliflower, and non-acidic vegetables aids in balancing stomach acid and reducing symptoms.
- Whole grains: incorporating oats, brown rice, and quinoa furnishes fiber and nutrients without provoking acid reflux.
- Low-fat dairy: moderate consumption of skim milk, yogurt, and cheese offers essential nutrients without aggravating the condition.

Chapter 2

8 Weeks Meal Plan for Acid Reflux Relief

In this chapter, we delve into a comprehensive 8-week meal plan meticulously crafted for individuals grappling with acid reflux, or gastroesophageal reflux disease (GERD). This prevalent digestive disorder arises when stomach acid regurgitates into the esophagus, resulting in distressing symptoms such as heartburn, regurgitation, and chest pain. Recognizing the pivotal role of diet in managing acid reflux, this meal plan is strategically designed to aid individuals in alleviating symptoms and enhancing overall digestive health. It incorporates an array of low-acid and non-acidic foods, complemented by tips for effective portion control and strategic meal timing. By adhering to this meticulously curated meal plan, individuals can proactively take charge of their acid reflux, experiencing relief from the discomfort and pain often associated with this condition.

Week 1: Kickstarting Your Acid Reflux Diet

The inaugural week of the 8-week meal plan for acid reflux relief concentrates on initiating the dietary transformation and making nuanced adjustments to alleviate symptoms. The overarching objective during this week is to introduce specific dietary modifications aimed at reducing acid reflux flare-ups and mitigating discomfort.

Day 1:

Breakfast: Commence the day with a bowl of oatmeal adorned with sliced bananas and a drizzle of honey. Oatmeal, renowned for its low acidity, aids in absorbing excess stomach acid, while bananas, being a non-acidic fruit, offer a soothing effect on the digestive tract.

Lunch: Revel in a grilled chicken salad featuring mixed greens, cherry tomatoes, and a light vinaigrette dressing. Grilled chicken, being a lean protein, proves gentle on the stomach, and the mixed greens supply essential nutrients without provoking acid reflux.

Dinner: Craft a delectable baked salmon accompanied by steamed vegetables and quinoa. Salmon, a fatty fish abundant in omega-3 fatty acids, contributes to reducing inflammation in the digestive system. Simultaneously, steamed vegetables and quinoa, both low-acid and high-fiber options, foster digestive health.

Day 2:

Breakfast: Indulge in a Greek yogurt parfait embellished with granola and fresh berries. Greek yogurt, a non-acidic dairy option rich in probiotics, aids in digestion and supports gut health.

Lunch: Opt for a turkey and avocado wrap enveloped in a whole grain tortilla, accompanied by a side of mixed fruit. Turkey, as a lean protein, is less likely to trigger acid reflux, and the inclusion of avocado provides healthy fats beneficial for the digestive system.

Dinner: Prepare a vegetable stir-fry starring tofu and brown rice. Tofu, being a plant-based protein, proves gentle on the stomach, while brown rice, a low-acid and high-fiber alternative to white rice, promotes digestive well-being.

Day 3:

Breakfast: Savor a smoothie concocted with almond milk, spinach, pineapple, and a scoop of protein powder. Almond milk, a non-acidic dairy alternative, pairs harmoniously with spinach and pineapple, both alkaline-rich ingredients that aid in neutralizing stomach acid.

Lunch: Relish a quinoa salad featuring black beans, corn, cherry tomatoes, and a lime vinaigrette. Quinoa, black beans, and corn collectively present low-acid, high-fiber attributes conducive to digestive health.

Dinner: Prepare succulent grilled shrimp skewers complemented by roasted vegetables and a side of couscous. Shrimp, a lean protein less likely to trigger acid reflux, coupled with roasted vegetables, proves stomach-friendly while delivering essential nutrients.

Day 4:

Breakfast: Initiate the day with a slice of whole-grain toast adorned with almond butter and sliced strawberries. Whole grain toast, a low-acid option, harmonizes with the non-acidic, high-fiber choices of almond butter and strawberries to support digestive health.

Lunch: Opt for a tuna salad featuring mixed greens, cucumber, and a light citrus vinaigrette. Tuna, being a lean protein, demonstrates gentleness on the stomach, and the citrus vinaigrette incorporates alkaline-rich ingredients to alleviate acid reflux symptoms.

Dinner: Prepare a lean beef stir-fry incorporating mixed vegetables and brown rice. Lean beef, a low-acid protein choice, combined with mixed vegetables, imparts essential nutrients without aggravating acid reflux.

Day 5:

Breakfast: Partake in a bowl of low-acid, high-fiber cereal with almond milk and sliced peaches. Opt for a cereal low in sugar and high in fiber to fortify digestive health, coupling it with non-acidic almond milk and peaches.

Lunch: Revel in a grilled vegetable and hummus wrap, ensconced in a whole grain tortilla, accompanied by a side of fresh fruit. Grilled vegetables prove stomach-friendly, while hummus, being a non-acidic, high-fiber spread, supports digestive health.

Dinner: Craft a vegetarian chili featuring kidney beans, bell peppers, onions, and a side of whole-grain bread. Kidney beans, constituting a low-acid, high-fiber option, contribute to digestive health, while whole grain bread stands as a non-acidic, high-fiber choice.

Week 2: Incorporating Low-Acid Foods

As we transition into the second week of our meticulously designed 8-week meal plan for acid reflux relief, the spotlight turns towards seamlessly integrating an array of low-acid and non-acidic foods into the diet. This strategic shift aims to empower individuals in proactively managing their symptoms while fostering improvements in overall digestive health. By consciously opting for foods and beverages less likely to trigger acid reflux, participants can embark on a journey toward enhanced well-being.

Day 1:

Breakfast: Initiate the day with a revitalizing smoothie crafted from almond milk, spinach, banana, and a scoop of protein powder. Almond milk, a non-acidic dairy alternative, harmonizes with the alkaline-rich attributes of spinach and banana, collectively contributing to neutralizing stomach acid.

Lunch: Relish a grilled chicken Caesar salad featuring romaine lettuce, grilled chicken breast, and a light Caesar dressing. Romaine lettuce, chosen for its low acidity, aligns seamlessly with grilled chicken, a lean protein that proves gentle on the stomach.

Dinner: Indulge in the flavors of baked cod complemented by roasted sweet potatoes and a side of quinoa. Cod, a lean and white fish, stands as a choice less likely to trigger acid reflux, while sweet potatoes and quinoa, both low-acid and high-fiber selections, actively promote digestive health.

Day 2:

Breakfast: Savor a bowl of low-acid, high-fiber cereal paired with almond milk and mixed berries. Choosing a cereal low in sugar and high in fiber fosters digestive health, complemented by the non-acidic nature of almond milk and the berry ensemble.

Lunch: Opt for a turkey and cranberry wrap enclosed in a whole grain tortilla, accompanied by a side of mixed green salad. Turkey, recognized for being a lean protein less likely to trigger acid reflux, pairs harmoniously with cranberries, non-acidic fruits known for their digestive soothing properties.

Dinner: Delight in a grilled vegetable and quinoa salad adorned with a light balsamic vinaigrette. Grilled vegetables, gentle on the stomach, seamlessly combine with quinoa, a low-acid, high-fiber alternative to other grains.

Day 3:

Breakfast: Relish a Greek yogurt parfait enriched with granola and sliced peaches. Greek yogurt, a non-acidic dairy option replete with probiotics, contributes to digestive health, and peaches, being non-acidic and high-fiber, further enhance the fruitfulness of this morning's delight.

Lunch: Indulge in a tuna salad featuring mixed greens, cherry tomatoes, and a light citrus vinaigrette. Tuna, selected for its status as a gentle lean protein, aligns with a citrus vinaigrette containing alkaline-rich ingredients, effectively mitigating acid reflux symptoms.

Dinner: Embark on a culinary journey with a vegetarian stir-fry showcasing tofu and brown rice. Tofu, a plant-based protein renowned for its stomach-friendly nature, finds synergy with brown rice, a low-acid and high-fiber alternative to its refined counterpart.

Day 4:

Breakfast: Begin the day anew with a revitalizing smoothie featuring almond milk, kale, pineapple, and a scoop of protein powder. Almond milk, reiterating its non-acidic dairy alternative status, harmonizes with kale and pineapple, both possessing alkaline-rich attributes that aid in neutralizing stomach acid.

Lunch: Revisit the delightful flavors of a grilled chicken Caesar salad, this time featuring romaine lettuce, grilled chicken breast, and a light Caesar dressing. Romaine lettuce and grilled chicken once again grace the palate as a delightful, low-acid combination.

Dinner: Savor the richness of grilled salmon partnered with asparagus and a side of quinoa.

Salmon, a fatty fish teeming with omega-3 fatty acids, boasts anti-inflammatory properties beneficial for digestive health. Accompanied by asparagus and quinoa, both low-acid and high-fiber selections, this dish stands as a testament to fostering digestive well-being.

Day 5:

Breakfast: Partake in a comforting bowl of oatmeal crowned with almond butter and sliced bananas. Oatmeal, celebrated for its low-acid profile, adeptly absorbs excess stomach acid, while almond butter and bananas, both non-acidic and high-fiber choices, further contribute to supporting digestive health.

Lunch: Delight in a turkey and avocado wrap, enveloped in a whole grain tortilla, alongside a side of mixed fruit. Turkey, recognized for its lean protein attributes, teams up with avocado, offering healthy fats beneficial for the digestive system.

Dinner: Conclude the week with a delectable vegetable and tofu stir-fry, accompanied by brown rice. Tofu, celebrated for its plant-based protein and gentle impact on the stomach, combines seamlessly with brown rice, a low-acid, high-fiber alternative to its refined counterpart.

Week 3: Introducing Anti-Inflammatory Ingredients

As we step into the third week of our thoughtfully crafted meal plan for acid reflux relief, our primary focus shifts toward the integration of potent anti-inflammatory ingredients. The objective is to harness the potential of these ingredients to alleviate inflammation in the digestive tract, thereby providing much-needed relief from acid reflux symptoms. By incorporating these elements into your meals, we aim to create a soothing effect on the esophageal lining, ultimately reducing the discomfort associated with acid reflux.

Ginger:

A pivotal anti-inflammatory addition to our Week 3 meal plan is ginger. Revered for its anti-inflammatory properties, ginger has been a staple in traditional medicine for centuries, renowned for aiding digestion and alleviating stomach discomfort. Introducing fresh ginger into dishes like stir-fries, soups, and teas offers a flavorful approach to relieving acid reflux symptoms.

Turmeric:

Another formidable anti-inflammatory contender making its way into the Week 3 repertoire is turmeric. Curcumin, the active compound in turmeric, boasts both anti-inflammatory and antioxidant properties. Scientifically proven to alleviate symptoms of acid reflux, turmeric becomes a versatile addition to dishes such as curries, stews, and smoothies, contributing to the reduction of inflammation and discomfort.

Additional Anti-Inflammatory Ingredients:

Week 3 doesn't solely revolve around ginger and turmeric; it introduces a medley of other anti-inflammatory ingredients to enhance the meal plan's efficacy. Garlic, renowned for its culinary versatility, joins the lineup, accompanied by the wholesome goodness of leafy greens and omega-3-rich fatty fish. Together, these ingredients work synergistically to diminish inflammation in the digestive tract, providing tangible relief from acid reflux symptoms.

In the third week of our meal plan, the breakfast, snack, lunch, snack, and dinner selections are meticulously curated to seamlessly incorporate these anti-inflammatory ingredients, creating a holistic approach to alleviate the discomfort associated with acid reflux.

Breakfast:
Commence your day with a comforting bowl of oatmeal adorned with fresh berries and a sprinkle of chia seeds. Oats, rich in fiber, and berries, abundant in antioxidants, form a powerhouse duo combating inflammation in the body. This breakfast not only satisfies your taste buds but also sets the tone for an anti-inflammatory start to the day.

Snack:
For a mid-morning snack, indulge in a handful of raw almonds or walnuts. These nutrient-packed nuts offer a delightful combination of anti-inflammatory compounds and healthy fats, contributing to the reduction of inflammation and ensuring a satisfying snack experience.

Lunch:

At midday, opt for a vibrant and nutrient-dense salad featuring spinach, kale, and other leafy greens. Top it with grilled salmon or chickpeas to introduce omega-3 fatty acids and protein—both revered for their anti-inflammatory prowess. This lunch choice not only tantalizes the taste buds but also nourishes the body with elements known to alleviate inflammation.

Snack:

Choose a refreshing green smoothie for your afternoon snack, blending kale, cucumber, ginger, and pineapple. Green vegetables and ginger bring their anti-inflammatory effects to the mix, while pineapple introduces bromelain—an enzyme recognized for its ability to reduce inflammation and aid digestion.

Dinner:

Cap off the day with a comforting bowl of quinoa and vegetable stir-fry. Packed with colorful vegetables like bell peppers, broccoli, and carrots, and featuring quinoa—a gluten-free whole grain rich in anti-inflammatory compounds—this dinner option not only delights the palate but also supports overall health and well-being through its anti-inflammatory properties.

Week 4: Balancing pH Levels with Alkaline Foods

As we delve into the fourth week of our carefully structured meal plan for acid reflux relief, our attention shifts towards the crucial objective of balancing pH levels through the incorporation of alkaline foods. Often, acid reflux stems from an imbalance in the body's pH levels, where an excess of acidic foods contributes to heightened acidity in the stomach and digestive tract. By introducing alkaline foods into our diet, we aim to restore equilibrium to the body's pH levels, subsequently alleviating the symptoms associated with acid reflux.

Key Alkaline Foods:

Week 4 strategically integrates key alkaline foods to counteract the acidic imbalance. Leafy greens, including spinach, kale, and Swiss chard, take center stage. These highly alkaline vegetables play a pivotal role in neutralizing stomach acidity when incorporated into salads, smoothies, and stir-fries.

Additionally, root vegetables, such as sweet potatoes, carrots, and beets, make a significant appearance in the Week 4 meal plan. Laden with alkalinity, these vegetables become valuable allies in neutralizing stomach acid when enjoyed in roasted dishes, soups, and stews.

Alkaline-Rich Menu:

In addition to leafy greens and root vegetables, Week 4 introduces other alkaline-rich foods such as almonds, tofu, and quinoa. These components are strategically chosen to rebalance the body's pH levels and provide much-needed relief from acid reflux symptoms.

To further enhance the alkaline-rich experience, the breakfast, snack, lunch, snack, and dinner selections are meticulously curated for optimal pH balance.

Breakfast:

Embark on your day with a revitalizing and alkalizing green smoothie crafted from spinach, cucumber, celery, and a splash of lemon juice. Green vegetables, renowned for their alkaline properties, are complemented by the acidic touch of lemon juice, working synergistically to alkalize the body.

Snack:

Indulge in a light and alkaline snack by munching on sliced cucumbers or carrot sticks paired with hummus. Both cucumbers and carrots are alkaline-forming foods, acting as effective counters to acidity in the body.

Lunch:

Delight in a vibrant salad featuring mixed greens, avocado, and a choice of grilled chicken or tofu. Avocado, a highly alkaline fruit, contributes to balancing pH levels and reducing overall acidity in the body.

Snack:

For a satisfying mid-afternoon snack, opt for a small serving of alkaline-rich almonds or pumpkin seeds. These nuts and seeds actively promote alkalinity in the body, aiding in the reduction of acidity.

Dinner:

Conclude the day with a nourishing and alkaline-rich meal—baked salmon accompanied by steamed asparagus and quinoa. Salmon, rich in omega-3 fatty acids with alkalizing properties, pairs seamlessly with asparagus and quinoa, both highly alkaline foods contributing to the restoration of pH balance in the body.

Week 5: Tailoring Your Diet to Combat Acid Reflux

As we step into Week 5 of our comprehensive 8-week meal plan, the spotlight shines on the critical aspect of customizing your diet to effectively manage the individual nuances of acid reflux symptoms. This segment places a robust emphasis on the identification of trigger foods, advocating for necessary adjustments tailored to individual needs. The primary objective is to curate a diet that eliminates or reduces the intake of foods and beverages known to exacerbate acid reflux symptoms, including spicy foods, citrus fruits, chocolate, caffeine, and alcohol.

A central tenet of Week 5 involves the incorporation of a diverse array of low-acid foods, strategically selected to be gentle on the stomach while delivering essential nutrients that support overall health and well-being. The meal plan features an extensive repertoire of recipes, thoughtfully crafted to include these low-acid foods, offering individuals a delightful variety of satisfying meal options devoid of exacerbating acid reflux symptoms.

Beyond the focus on low-acid foods, Week 5 underscores the significance of two essential factors: portion control and mindful eating. Acknowledging that overeating can exert undue pressure on the stomach, leading to acid reflux symptoms, this week encourages individuals to adopt a mindful approach to portion sizes. By savoring each bite and consuming meals slowly, individuals can effectively manage their symptoms and promote optimal digestive health.

Moreover, Week 5 advocates for heightened awareness regarding post-meal experiences and introduces the practice of maintaining a food journal. This proactive measure allows individuals to systematically track their symptoms, enabling the identification of specific trigger foods. Armed with this knowledge, individuals can make informed dietary choices, steering clear of foods that intensify acid reflux symptoms.

In essence, Week 5 empowers individuals to take charge of their acid reflux by providing practical tools for customization. By tailoring their diet, being mindful of portions, and maintaining a vigilant eye on symptom triggers, individuals can not only manage but also gain mastery over their acid reflux, fostering a path towards improved digestive health and overall well-being.

Week 6: Enhancing Digestive Wellness with Probiotic-Rich Foods

As we venture into Week 6 of our meticulously crafted 8-week meal plan, our focus converges on the pivotal role of integrating probiotic foods into the diet. This strategic emphasis aims to champion digestive health and assuage the symptoms associated with acid reflux. Probiotics, revered as beneficial bacteria, wield the power to reinstate equilibrium in the gut microbiota, ushering in an era of improved digestion. The inclusion of probiotic-rich foods becomes instrumental in fostering the growth of healthy bacteria within the gut, mitigating inflammation, and ultimately culminating in enhanced digestive function and diminished manifestations of acid reflux.

Week 6 unfolds a carefully curated meal plan featuring an array of recipes that showcase probiotic-rich ingredients. From yogurt and kefir to miso, kimchi, and sauerkraut, these foods not only serve as rich sources of essential probiotics but also stand as nutritional powerhouses offering a spectrum of nutrients vital for overall health. By seamlessly incorporating these probiotic-rich foods into their diet, individuals embark on a journey to cultivate a flourishing gut microbiota, subsequently elevating their digestive health. The outcome is a reduction in acid reflux symptoms, coupled with an overall improvement in well-being.

In tandem with the focus on probiotic-rich foods, Week 6 underscores the paramount importance of maintaining a well-rounded and diverse diet. This entails the inclusion of an assortment of fruits, vegetables, whole grains, and lean proteins—providing the necessary nutrients crucial for sustaining digestive health. By diversifying their food intake, individuals can ensure a holistic supply of nutrients, contributing to the fortification of overall health and well-being.

Moreover, Week 6 of the meal plan extends its guidance beyond dietary considerations, advocating for the adoption of healthy lifestyle habits that further fortify digestive health. Hydration, regular exercise, and stress management take center stage in this holistic approach. By incorporating these positive habits into their daily routine, individuals can amplify the support for their digestive health, paving the way for a reduction in acid reflux symptoms and an enhanced state of overall well-being.

Week 7: Embracing Plant-Based Solutions for Acid Reflux Relief

As we embark on the seventh week of our comprehensive meal plan, our attention shifts towards exploring plant-based alternatives tailored for individuals grappling with acid reflux.

Plant-based diets have emerged as a beneficial choice for those with GERD, owing to their high fiber content and lower fat composition. These diets not only foster overall digestive health but also hold the potential to assuage the symptoms associated with acid reflux. Let's delve into guidelines and tantalizing plant-based meal options designed to manage acid reflux effectively:

1. Breakfast:
- Overnight oats featuring almond milk, chia seeds, and a medley of fresh berries.
- Whole grain toast adorned with creamy avocado slices and succulent tomatoes.
- A rejuvenating smoothie concocted with spinach, banana, almond milk, and a touch of protein powder.

2. Lunch:
- Quinoa salad boasting an array of vibrant vegetables, dressed in a zesty lemon vinaigrette.
- Wholesome black bean and corn tacos embraced by whole grain tortillas.
- A hearty serving of lentil soup complemented by a side of mixed greens.

3. Dinner:

- Delectable stuffed bell peppers generously filled with quinoa, black beans, and aromatic spices.
- Eggplant and chickpea curry, lovingly served with a bed of nourishing brown rice.
- Flavorful Portobello mushroom burgers, accompanied by crispy sweet potato fries.

4. Snacks:

- A nutrient-rich mix of assorted nuts and seeds.
- Fresh, vibrant fruit slices paired with luscious almond butter.
- Hummus served alongside crisp vegetable sticks for a satisfying crunch.

While transitioning to a plant-based diet can significantly impact acid reflux management, it is crucial to ensure meals are well-balanced, providing all essential nutrients. Additionally, paying attention to portion sizes and steering clear of trigger foods like citrus fruits, tomatoes, and spicy dishes remains pivotal.

Week 8: Sustaining Your Acid Reflux Diet

As we gracefully approach the final week of our curated meal plan, the spotlight now turns to sustaining the acid reflux diet in the long term. While the 8-week meal plan provides a structured roadmap for managing acid reflux, the journey extends beyond this timeframe, demanding continued dietary choices that champion digestive health and mitigate the risk of acid reflux symptoms. Here are some enduring tips for sustaining the acid reflux diet:

1. Be Mindful of Trigger Foods:
   - Continued vigilance towards trigger foods is paramount in minimizing the recurrence of acid reflux episodes. Steering clear of citrus fruits, tomatoes, chocolate, fatty/fried foods, and caffeine remains an integral part of long-term management.

2. Portion Control:
   - Maintaining portion control is an enduring cornerstone for sustaining the acid reflux diet. By adopting a habit of consuming smaller, more frequent meals, individuals can thwart overeating and effectively manage their acid reflux.

3. Stay Hydrated:

- Adequate hydration is a perpetual necessity for supporting digestive health and curbing acid reflux symptoms. Diluting stomach acid and facilitating proper digestion, it is advised to consume at least 8-10 cups of water daily.

4. Incorporate Regular Exercise:

- Regular physical activity, persistently woven into the routine, can contribute to managing acid reflux by fostering healthy digestion and maintaining an optimal weight. Exercise aids in strengthening the lower esophageal sphincter, preventing the backward flow of stomach acid.

5. Seek Professional Guidance:

- For those contending with chronic or severe acid reflux, seeking ongoing professional guidance from healthcare providers or registered dietitians remains indispensable. These experts can offer personalized recommendations and steadfast support, ensuring the continued management of acid reflux through tailored dietary and lifestyle adjustments.

Chapter 3

Comprehensive List of 100 Recipes to Help Improve Acid Reflux Health

Acid reflux, also known as gastroesophageal reflux disease (GERD), is a common condition that affects millions of people worldwide. It occurs when the stomach acid flows back into the esophagus, causing a burning sensation in the chest and throat. While medications can help manage the symptoms of acid reflux, dietary changes can also play a significant role in alleviating the discomfort associated with the condition.

In this chapter, we will provide a comprehensive list of 100 recipes specifically designed to help improve acid reflux health. These recipes focus on using ingredients that are gentle on the digestive system and are less likely to trigger acid reflux symptoms. Whether you're looking for breakfast options, lunch ideas, dinner recipes, or snacks and desserts, you'll find a variety of delicious and reflux-friendly options to suit your taste and dietary preferences.

Breakfast Options

1. Oatmeal with Almond Milk and Bananas

Ingredients:
- 1 cup rolled oats
- 2 cups almond milk
- 2 ripe bananas, sliced
- 1 tablespoon honey (optional)
- 1 teaspoon cinnamon
- 1/4 cup chopped almonds
- Pinch of salt

Instructions:

1. In a medium saucepan, bring the almond milk to a simmer over medium heat.

2. Once the almond milk is simmering, stir in the rolled oats and a pinch of salt. Reduce the heat to low and let the oatmeal cook for about 10-15 minutes, stirring occasionally, until the oatmeal reaches your desired consistency.

3. While the oatmeal is cooking, slice the bananas and chop the almonds.

4. Once the oatmeal is ready, remove the saucepan from the heat and stir in the honey (if using) and cinnamon.

5. Divide the oatmeal into bowls and top each bowl with sliced bananas and chopped almonds.

6. Serve the oatmeal with almond milk and bananas warm and enjoy!

2. Greek Yogurt Parfait with Berries and Honey

Ingredients:

- 1 cup of Greek yogurt
- 1 cup of mixed berries (strawberries, blueberries, raspberries)
- 2 tablespoons of honey
- 1/4 cup of granola
- Fresh mint leaves for garnish (optional)

Instructions:

1. Start by washing and preparing the berries. Slice the strawberries and set aside.

2. In a small bowl, mix the Greek yogurt with 1 tablespoon of honey until well combined.

3. In serving glasses or bowls, begin layering the parfait. Start with a spoonful of the Greek yogurt, followed by a layer of mixed berries, then a sprinkle of granola.

4. Continue layering until the glasses are filled, ending with a dollop of Greek yogurt on top.

5. Drizzle the remaining honey over the parfaits for a touch of sweetness.

6. Garnish with fresh mint leaves if desired.

7. Serve the Greek yogurt parfaits immediately, or refrigerate for up to 2 hours before serving for a chilled treat.

3. Quinoa Breakfast Bowl with Fresh Fruit

Ingredients:
- 1 cup of quinoa
- 2 cups of water
- 1 teaspoon of cinnamon
- 1 teaspoon of vanilla extract
- 2 tablespoons of honey
- Fresh fruit (such as berries, bananas, or mango)
- Nuts or seeds for topping (such as almonds, walnuts, or chia seeds)
- Milk or yogurt (optional, for serving)

Instructions:

1. Rinse the quinoa under cold water using a fine mesh sieve to remove any bitterness.

2. In a medium-sized saucepan, add the rinsed quinoa and 2 cups of water. Bring to a boil over medium-high heat.

3. Once boiling, reduce the heat to low and let the quinoa simmer for about 15-20 minutes or until all the water is absorbed and the quinoa is light and fluffy.

4. Once the quinoa is cooked, remove it from the heat and stir in the cinnamon, vanilla extract, and honey.

5. Allow the quinoa to cool for a few minutes.

6. While the quinoa is cooling, prepare your choice of fresh fruit by washing and chopping it into bite-sized pieces.

7. Once the quinoa has cooled slightly, scoop it into a bowl and top with the fresh fruit.

8. Optionally, you can drizzle some milk or spoon some yogurt over the top for added creaminess.

9. Finally, sprinkle some nuts or seeds over the top for a crunchy texture and added nutrition.

10. Enjoy your delicious and nutritious quinoa breakfast bowl with fresh fruit!

Other Breakfast options Include:

4. Avocado Toast with Whole Grain Bread
5. Spinach and Feta Omelet
6. Chia Seed Pudding with Coconut Milk
7. Buckwheat Pancakes with Maple Syrup
8. Smoothie Bowl with Spinach, Pineapple, and Coconut Water
9. Scrambled Eggs with Low-Fat Cheese and Vegetables
10. Whole Grain Toast with Almond Butter and Sliced Apples
11. Baked Sweet Potato Hash with Eggs
12. Cottage Cheese and Fruit Salad
13. Breakfast Burrito with Black Beans and Avocado
14. Quinoa and Veggie Breakfast Muffins
15. Brown Rice Congee with Ginger and Scallions
16. Cinnamon Raisin French Toast with Berries
17. Chia Seed and Berry Smoothie
18. Spinach and Mushroom Frittata
19. Whole Grain Waffle with Fresh Strawberries
20. Overnight Chia Seed Pudding with Mango and Coconut Flakes

Lunch Ideas

1. Quinoa Salad with Grilled Chicken and Veggies

Ingredients:
- 1 cup of quinoa
- 2 cups of water
- 2 boneless, skinless chicken breasts
- 1 medium red bell pepper, diced
- 1 medium yellow bell pepper, diced
- 1 small red onion, thinly sliced
- 1 cup of cherry tomatoes, halved
- 1/4 cup of fresh parsley, chopped
- 1/4 cup of olive oil
- 2 tablespoons of balsamic vinegar
- 1 tablespoon of Dijon mustard
- Salt and pepper to taste

Instructions:

1. Start by cooking the quinoa. In a medium saucepan, combine the quinoa and water. Bring to a boil, then reduce heat to low and simmer for about 15 minutes, or until all the water has been absorbed. Remove from heat and let it cool.

2. While the quinoa is cooking, prepare the chicken. Season the chicken breasts with salt and pepper, then grill them over medium-high heat for about 6-7 minutes on each side, or until they are fully cooked. Let them cool, then slice them into strips.

3. In a large bowl, combine the cooked quinoa, grilled chicken, diced bell peppers, sliced red onion, cherry tomatoes, and chopped parsley.

4. In a small bowl, whisk together the olive oil, balsamic vinegar, Dijon mustard, salt, and pepper. Pour this dressing over the quinoa and chicken mixture, and toss everything together until well combined.

5. Serve the quinoa salad immediately, or refrigerate it for a few hours to allow the flavors to meld together. Enjoy!

2. Turkey and Avocado Wrap with Whole Wheat Tortilla

Ingredients:
- 4 whole wheat tortillas
- 1 lb sliced turkey
- 1 ripe avocado, sliced
- 1 cup shredded lettuce
- 1/2 cup diced tomatoes
- 1/4 cup diced red onions
- 1/4 cup sliced black olives
- 1/2 cup shredded cheddar cheese
- 1/4 cup plain Greek yogurt
- 2 tbsp ranch dressing
- Salt and pepper to taste

Instructions:
1. Lay out the whole wheat tortillas on a clean surface.
2. In a small bowl, mix together the Greek yogurt and ranch dressing until well combined. Set aside.
3. Place a layer of sliced turkey on each tortilla, leaving about an inch of space on the edges.
4. Next, add a layer of sliced avocado on top of the turkey.

5. Sprinkle shredded lettuce, diced tomatoes, red onions, and black olives on top of the avocado.

6. Drizzle the Greek yogurt and ranch dressing mixture evenly over the ingredients on each tortilla.

7. Finally, sprinkle shredded cheddar cheese on top and season with salt and pepper to taste.

8. Carefully roll up each tortilla, folding in the sides as you go to keep the filling secure.

9. Use a sharp knife to slice each wrap in half diagonally for a clean presentation.

10. Serve the turkey and avocado wraps immediately, or wrap them in foil or plastic wrap for a convenient on-the-go meal.

3. Grilled Vegetable Panini with Pesto

Ingredients:
- 1 small zucchini, sliced
- 1 small yellow squash, sliced
- 1 red bell pepper, sliced
- 1 yellow bell pepper, sliced
- 1 small red onion, sliced

- 3 tablespoons olive oil
- Salt and pepper to taste
- 4 large ciabatta rolls, sliced in half
- 1/2 cup prepared pesto
- 8 slices mozzarella cheese
- 1 cup baby arugula

Instructions:

1. Preheat the grill to medium-high heat.
2. In a large mixing bowl, toss the zucchini, yellow squash, bell peppers, and red onion with olive oil. Season with salt and pepper.
3. Grill the vegetables for 3-4 minutes on each side, or until they have charred grill marks and are tender.
4. Once the vegetables are grilled, transfer them back to the mixing bowl and set aside.
5. Place the ciabatta rolls on the grill, cut side down, and toast for 1-2 minutes, until lightly golden brown.
6. Spread about a tablespoon of pesto on the bottom half of each ciabatta roll.
7. Layer the grilled vegetables on top of the pesto, followed by two slices of mozzarella cheese.
8. Top with a handful of baby arugula and place the remaining half of the ciabatta roll on top.
9. Place the assembled paninis back on the grill and press down with a spatula to help the cheese melt and the bread get nice grill marks.

10. Grill for 3-4 minutes on each side, or until the cheese is melted and the bread is crispy and golden brown.

11. Remove the paninis from the grill and let them rest for a few minutes before slicing and serving.

Other Lunch Options include:

4. Tuna Salad Lettuce Wraps

5. Lentil Soup with Spinach and Tomatoes

6. Chicken and Vegetable Stir-Fry with Brown Rice

7. Black Bean and Corn Quesadilla with Salsa

8. Mediterranean Chickpea Salad

9. Shrimp and Avocado Salad with Lemon Vinaigrette

10. Brown Rice Sushi Roll with Cucumber and Avocado

11. Roasted Vegetable Quinoa Bowl

12. Turkey and Hummus Sandwich on Whole Grain Bread

13. Veggie Burger with Lettuce and Tomato

14. Spinach and Strawberry Salad with Poppy Seed Dressing

15. Broccoli and Cheddar Soup

16. Grilled Salmon Salad with Citrus Vinaigrette

17. Egg Salad Wrap with Whole Wheat Tortilla

18. Quinoa and Black Bean Stuffed Peppers
19. Chicken and Kale Caesar Salad
20. Whole Wheat Pita with Greek Salad
21. Veggie and Brown Rice Wrap with Tahini Sauce
22. Roasted Red Pepper and Tomato Soup
23. Sesame Ginger Tofu Stir-Fry
24. Caprese Salad with Balsamic Glaze
25. Mexican Quinoa Salad with Avocado Dressing

Dinner Recipes

1. Lentil Curry with Cauliflower Rice Recipe

Ingredients:

- 1 cup of red lentils

- 1 head of cauliflower
- 1 onion, diced
- 2 cloves of garlic, minced
- 1 can of coconut milk
- 1 can of diced tomatoes
- 2 tbsp of curry powder
- 1 tsp of ground cumin
- 1 tsp of ground coriander
- 1 tsp of turmeric
- Salt and pepper to taste
- Fresh cilantro for garnish

Instructions:

1. Start by rinsing the red lentils in a fine-mesh strainer and set them aside.

2. Next, cut the cauliflower into florets and add them to a food processor. Pulse the cauliflower until it resembles the texture of rice. You can also use a grater to achieve the same result.

3. In a large skillet, heat a tablespoon of oil over medium heat. Add the diced onion and minced garlic to the skillet and sauté until the onion is translucent.

4. Once the onion and garlic are cooked, add the cauliflower rice to the skillet and sauté for 5-7 minutes until it becomes tender. Season with salt and pepper to taste and set the cauliflower rice aside.

5. In a large pot, add the rinsed red lentils, coconut milk, diced tomatoes, curry powder, cumin, coriander, turmeric, salt, and pepper. Stir everything together and bring the mixture to a boil.

6. Once the lentil mixture is boiling, reduce the heat to a simmer and let it cook for 20-25 minutes, or until the lentils are tender and the curry has thickened.

7. To serve, spoon the lentil curry over the cauliflower rice and garnish with fresh cilantro.

2. Baked Fish with Lemon and Dill

Ingredients:
- 4 fish fillets (such as cod or halibut)
- 4 tablespoons of melted butter
- 1 tablespoon of fresh lemon juice
- 2 cloves of minced garlic
- 2 tablespoons of freshly chopped dill
- Salt and pepper to taste
- Sliced lemon for garnish

Instructions:

1. Preheat your oven to 375°F (190°C), and lightly grease a baking dish with a little butter or cooking spray.

2. Place the fish fillets into the prepared baking dish, and brush them with the melted butter.

3. In a small bowl, mix together the lemon juice, minced garlic, and chopped dill. Evenly distribute this mixture over the fish fillets, and season them with salt and pepper.

4. Place slices of lemon on top of each fillet for added flavor and presentation.

5. Bake the fish in the preheated oven for 15-20 minutes, or until it easily flakes with a fork.

6. Once the fish is cooked through, carefully remove it from the oven and let it rest for a few minutes before serving.

3. Grilled Chicken with Quinoa Pilaf

Ingredients:
- 4 boneless, skinless chicken breasts
- 1 cup quinoa
- 2 cups chicken broth
- 1 small onion, diced
- 2 cloves garlic, minced
- 1 cup mixed vegetables (such as bell peppers, zucchini, and cherry tomatoes)
- 2 tablespoons olive oil
- 1 teaspoon dried oregano
- 1 teaspoon dried thyme
- Salt and pepper to taste

- Lemon wedges for serving

Instructions:

1. Start by preparing the quinoa pilaf. In a medium saucepan, heat 1 tablespoon of olive oil over medium heat. Add the diced onion and minced garlic and sauté for 2-3 minutes until the onion is translucent.

2. Add the quinoa to the saucepan and toast it for 2-3 minutes, stirring constantly. This will enhance the nutty flavor of the quinoa.

3. Pour in the chicken broth and bring it to a boil. Once boiling, reduce the heat to low, cover the saucepan, and let the quinoa simmer for 15-20 minutes, or until all the liquid has been absorbed and the quinoa is tender.

4. While the quinoa is cooking, preheat your grill to medium-high heat. Season the chicken breasts with dried oregano, dried thyme, salt, and pepper.

5. Grill the chicken for 6-7 minutes on each side, or until the internal temperature reaches 165°F. Cooking time may vary depending on the thickness of the chicken breasts.

6. While the chicken is cooking, toss the mixed vegetables with the remaining tablespoon of olive oil and season with salt and pepper. Grill the vegetables for 3-4 minutes, or until they are slightly charred and tender.

7. Once the quinoa is ready, fluff it with a fork and stir in the grilled vegetables.

8. Serve the grilled chicken on top of the quinoa pilaf and garnish with lemon wedges.

Other Dinner Options Include:

4. Eggplant and Mozzarella Stacks with Fresh Basil
5. Beef and Broccoli Stir-Fry with Brown Rice
6. Mushroom and Spinach Stuffed Chicken Breast
7. Turkey Meatballs with Marinara Sauce and Spaghetti Squash
8. Ginger and Garlic Glazed Salmon
9. Cauliflower Crust Pizza with Fresh Vegetables
10. Black Bean and Corn Stuffed Sweet Potatoes
11. Tofu and Vegetable Pad Thai
12. Spaghetti with Turkey Bolognese Sauce

13. Quinoa and Veggie Stuffed Portobello Mushrooms
14. Balsamic Glazed Chicken with Roasted Vegetables
15. Shrimp and Zucchini Noodles with Pesto
16. Vegan Lentil Shepherd's Pie
17. Grilled Steak with Chimichurri Sauce
18. Spinach and Artichoke Stuffed Chicken Breast
19. Veggie and Tofu Stir-Fry with Brown Rice
20. Quinoa and Black Bean Enchilada Bake
21. Lemon Herb Roasted Chicken with Quinoa
22. Ratatouille with Herbed Quinoa
23. Spicy Turkey Chili with Cornbread
24. Salmon Nicoise Salad
25. Coconut Curry Chicken with Cauliflower Rice

Snacks and Desserts

1. Cucumber and Hummus Slices

Ingredients:
- 1 large cucumber
- 1 cup of hummus
- 1 tablespoon of olive oil
- 1 teaspoon of paprika
- Salt and pepper to taste
- Fresh parsley for garnish

Instructions:
1. Start by washing the cucumber and patting it dry with a paper towel.
2. Cut off the ends of the cucumber and then slice it into thin rounds, about 1/4 inch thick.
3. Lay the cucumber slices on a serving platter in a single layer.

4. Next, scoop the hummus into a small bowl and add in the olive oil, paprika, salt, and pepper.

5. Stir the ingredients together until well combined.

6. Using a small spoon or knife, spread a dollop of the hummus mixture onto each cucumber slice, covering the entire surface.

7. Once all the cucumber slices are topped with hummus, sprinkle some freshly chopped parsley over the top for a pop of color and flavor.

8. Serve the cucumber and hummus slices immediately, or cover and refrigerate for later.

2. Apple Slices with Almond Butter

Ingredients:
- 2 apples, sliced
- 1/4 cup almond butter
- 1 tablespoon honey
- 1 teaspoon cinnamon
- 1/4 cup sliced almonds

Instructions:

1. Wash the apples and slice them into thin, even pieces. Place them on a serving platter or individual plates.

2. In a small bowl, mix together the almond butter, honey, and cinnamon until well combined.

3. Using a butter knife or spoon, spread a generous amount of the almond butter mixture onto each apple slice.

4. Sprinkle the sliced almonds over the top of the almond butter.

5. Serve immediately and enjoy!

3. Greek Yogurt with Berries and Granola

Ingredients:

- 1 cup of Greek yogurt
- 1/2 cup of mixed berries (strawberries, blueberries, raspberries)
- 1/4 cup of granola
- 1 tablespoon of honey
- 1 teaspoon of chia seeds

Instructions :

1. Start by choosing a good quality Greek yogurt. Greek yogurt is thick, creamy and has a slightly tangy flavor, which pairs perfectly with the sweetness of the berries and granola.

2. Pour the Greek yogurt into a bowl or serving dish. Make sure to use a generous portion as the yogurt will act as the base for the rest of the ingredients.

3. Wash the berries and pat them dry with a paper towel. Cut any large berries, like strawberries, into smaller pieces if desired.

4. Sprinkle the berries over the Greek yogurt, distributing them evenly to ensure each spoonful contains a variety of flavors.

5. Next, add the granola on top of the berries. Granola adds a satisfying crunch and a toasty flavor to the dish. It also provides a good source of fiber and nutrients.

6. Drizzle the honey over the yogurt, berries, and granola. The honey will add a natural sweetness and a pleasant aroma to the dish.

7. Lastly, sprinkle the chia seeds over the top. Chia seeds are high in omega-3 fatty acids, fiber, and protein, making them a nutritious addition to the dish.

8. Serve immediately and enjoy your delicious and nutritious Greek yogurt with berries and granola. This dish is perfect for breakfast, a snack, or even as a light dessert. It provides a balance of creamy, crunchy, sweet, and tangy flavors that will leave you feeling satisfied and nourished.

Other Snacks and Desserts Options Include:

4. Trail Mix with Nuts and Dried Fruit
5. Rice Cake with Peanut Butter and Sliced Banana
6. Roasted Chickpeas with Chili and Lime
7. Mixed Berries with Dark Chocolate Drizzle
8. Carrot Sticks with Greek Yogurt Ranch Dip
9. Homemade Popcorn with Nutritional Yeast
10. Chia Seed Pudding with Mango and Coconut Flakes
11. Baked Apple Chips with Cinnamon
12. Frozen Grapes
13. Almond and Date Energy Bites
14. Mango and Pineapple Fruit Salad
15. Whole Grain Crackers with Avocado and Tomato Slices
16. Greek Yogurt Popsicles with Fresh Fruit
17. Berry Smoothie Bowl
18. Dark Chocolate and Almond Clusters
19. Pineapple and Coconut Sorbet
20. Mango and Banana Nice Cream
21. Almond Flour Banana Bread
22. Oatmeal and Raisin Cookies
23. Pecan and Maple Granola Bars
24. Strawberry and Coconut Yogurt Parfait
25. Grilled Peaches with Honey and Cinnamon

Chapter 4

Recognizing Foods to Steer Clear of for Acid Reflux Comfort

Acid reflux, commonly known as heartburn, stands as a persistent and discomforting condition impacting millions globally. Amidst the array of treatments and lifestyle modifications aiding symptom management, a pivotal aspect in thwarting flare-ups involves pinpointing and steering clear of specific trigger foods capable of exacerbating the condition.

This chapter undertakes an exploration of several common dietary culprits—ranging from high-fat and spicy to citrusy, caffeinated, chocolaty, alcoholic, processed, and sugary options—that can contribute to acid reflux. Moreover, we'll offer suitable alternatives catering to those grappling with this challenging condition.

High-Fat Foods:

High-fat foods emerge as frequent culprits triggering acid reflux due to their potential to relax the lower esophageal sphincter (LES). This vital muscular barrier, separating the stomach and the esophagus, tends to slacken when exposed to saturated fats found in fried foods, fatty meats, and full-fat dairy products. Mitigating acid reflux involves limiting the intake of these foods and opting for healthier, lower-fat alternatives like lean meats, low-fat dairy, and heart-healthy cooking oils such as olive or avocado oil.

Spicy Foods:

Especially seasoned with chili peppers, hot sauces, and other piquant ingredients, spicy foods can aggravate the esophagus and heighten acid reflux symptoms. Those contending with acid reflux are advised to steer clear of such culinary choices and instead gravitate towards milder seasonings and herbs for flavor enhancement.

Citrus Fruits:

Despite being rich in vitamins and antioxidants, citrus fruits like oranges, grapefruits, lemons, and limes can trigger acid reflux symptoms due to their high acidity. Managing acid reflux involves limiting the consumption of these fruits and opting for alternatives with lower acidity levels, such as apples, pears, and bananas.

Caffeine and Carbonated Drinks:

Recognized as a known trigger, caffeine can relax the LES and boost stomach acid production, making coffee, tea, and caffeinated sodas potential contributors to heightened symptoms. Carbonated drinks, too, can induce bloating and increase LES pressure. Advisable for those with acid reflux is to reduce or eliminate caffeine and carbonated beverages, opting instead for caffeine-free alternatives like herbal teas or water.

Chocolate and Mint:

Both chocolate and mint are acknowledged triggers for acid reflux symptoms. Chocolate contains caffeine and theobromine, relaxing the LES, while mint can worsen symptoms by relaxing esophageal muscles. Individuals managing acid reflux should limit the consumption of chocolate and mint-flavored products, opting for alternative treats less likely to induce symptoms.

Alcohol:

Alcohol can elevate stomach acid production and relax the LES, establishing it as a common acid reflux trigger. While indulging in moderation is an option, selecting lower-alcohol alternatives such as light beer or wine spritzers is recommended for those with acid reflux.

Processed Foods and Sugary Treats:

Processed foods and sugary treats, laden with fat, sugar, and other potential triggers, can exacerbate acid reflux symptoms. Opting for whole, unprocessed foods and curbing the intake of sugary treats proves instrumental in effectively managing acid reflux symptoms.

Discovering Suitable Alternatives:
Effectively managing acid reflux symptoms necessitates uncovering suitable alternatives to the aforementioned trigger foods. This involves integrating more fruits and vegetables, selecting lean meats, favoring whole grains over refined carbohydrates, and opting for low-fat or dairy-free alternatives. Exploring diverse cooking techniques and flavor profiles adds an enjoyable dimension to meals while ensuring they remain friendly to those grappling with acid reflux symptoms.

Chapter 5

Culinary Insights for Acid Reflux Alleviation

Acid reflux, or heartburn, is a prevalent digestive ailment wherein stomach acid ascends into the esophagus, resulting in discomfort and a burning sensation. For many, it's a chronic concern that necessitates dietary adjustments to circumvent triggering symptoms. This chapter delves into culinary strategies tailored explicitly for acid reflux sufferers, encompassing the utilization of herbs and spices for flavor sans triggers, optimal meal preparation techniques to facilitate digestion, the importance of portion control and mindful eating, and stress management practices to alleviate acid reflux symptoms.

Employing Herbs and Spices for Flavor without Triggers

1. Reflux-Friendly Herb and Spice Selection:
Some herbs and spices are more amicable to acid reflux sufferers. Ginger, renowned for its anti-inflammatory properties, can soothe the digestive system, making it an excellent choice. Other reflux-friendly options include fennel, turmeric, and oregano, infusing dishes with flavor minus the discomfort.

2. Flavor Experimentation:
Restricting certain herbs and spices need not equate to a flavorless culinary experience. Experimenting with alternative combinations allows acid reflux sufferers to relish delicious meals. For instance, a blend of parsley, basil, and thyme can impart freshness and vibrancy without triggering discomfort.

3. Incorporating Natural Flavorings:
Beyond herbs and spices, acid reflux sufferers can introduce natural flavorings such as citrus zest, garlic-infused oils, and vinegar-free dressings. These additions contribute depth and complexity to

dishes, offering a unique twist without provoking common reflux triggers.

Meal Preparation Techniques for Optimal Digestion

1. Avoiding Aggravating Cooking Methods:

Certain cooking methods, like frying and deep-frying, can yield heavy, greasy foods challenging for the digestive system. Opting for healthier alternatives such as baking, steaming, and grilling produces lighter, more easily digestible meals, diminishing the risk of acid reflux symptoms.

2. Discerning Ingredient Choices:

Ingredients significantly influence digestion. Opting for fresh, whole ingredients while steering clear of processed and high-fat foods is crucial. Lean proteins like poultry and fish, fruits, vegetables, whole grains, and low-fat dairy become go-to choices, fostering nourishment and easy digestion.

3. Portion Control:

Overeating compounds acid reflux symptoms by exerting pressure on the stomach, causing acid to flow back into the esophagus. Smaller, more frequent meals throughout the day, as opposed to larger ones, avert digestive overload, curbing discomfort and symptoms.

Portion Control and Mindful Eating

1. Visual Cues for Portion Control:

Portion control plays a pivotal role in acid reflux management. Employing smaller plates and bowls provides visual cues that assist in regulating portion sizes, preventing overindulgence. Measuring out portions of high-acid foods further aids in tracking intake and sidestepping reflux triggers.

2. Mindful Eating Practices:

Mindful eating, focusing on taste, texture, and aroma, proves essential in acid reflux management. Savoring each bite, chewing food thoroughly, and adopting a deliberate pace during meals aid in gauging hunger and fullness, thwarting overeating, and mitigating the risk of acid reflux.

3. Incorporating Smaller, Frequent Meals:

Integrating smaller, more frequent meals into daily routines counters acid reflux symptoms. Consuming five to six small meals instead of three large ones prevents stomach overload, diminishing the likelihood of acid reflux incidents.

Stress Management for Reduced Acid Reflux Symptoms

1. Mindful Practices:

Stress, linked to various health issues, including acid reflux, amplifies symptoms by escalating stomach acid production and inducing esophageal sphincter relaxation. Mindful practices like meditation, deep breathing, and yoga emerge as effective stress management tools, heightening awareness and facilitating stress modulation.

2. Regular Exercise:

Exercise serves as a valuable stress mitigator. Engaging in activities like walking, swimming, or cycling for at least 30 minutes daily reduces stress hormones, fostering well-being. Regular physical activity proves beneficial not only for stress management but also for overall health improvement.

3. Creating a Calming Meal Environment:

Establishing a tranquil mealtime setting free from distractions, noise, and stress contributes to stress reduction and acid reflux prevention. Devoting time to enjoy meals without haste allows for relaxation and aids in digestion, minimizing stress-related acid reflux symptoms.

Chapter 6

Adopting a Comprehensive Approach to Wellness for Acid Reflux Relief

Acid reflux, also recognized as gastroesophageal reflux disease (GERD), is a prevalent digestive ailment affecting millions worldwide. This condition transpires when stomach acid regurgitates into the esophagus, resulting in discomfort such as heartburn, chest pain, and swallowing difficulties. While medical treatments exist, a holistic wellness strategy assumes a pivotal role in mitigating and alleviating acid reflux symptoms.

In this chapter, we will elucidate the significance of embracing a holistic wellness approach for acid reflux management. We will scrutinize the impact of physical activity, elucidate stress management techniques, delve into relaxation practices, and underscore the importance of quality sleep. By amalgamating these holistic wellness principles into your daily regimen, substantial relief from acid reflux symptoms can be achieved, concurrently enhancing your overall well-being.

The Role of Physical Activity in Acid Reflux Management

1. Benefits of Regular Exercise:

Regular physical activity stands out as a crucial player in acid reflux management. Scientific evidence indicates that moderate-intensity exercises like walking, swimming, and cycling contribute to diminished acid reflux occurrences. Exercise not only aids in weight management but also enhances digestion, mitigates stress, and fosters overall physical and mental well-being.

2. Weight Management:

Maintaining a healthy weight is pivotal in acid reflux control. Excess weight, especially around the abdomen, increases the risk of acid reflux by exerting pressure on the stomach. Regular physical activity assists in weight maintenance, reducing the severity of acid reflux symptoms.

3. Promoting Digestive Health:

Physical activity accelerates the movement of food through the digestive system, lowering the likelihood of acid reflux. Simultaneously, exercise is instrumental in stress reduction, a known catalyst for acid reflux. Engaging in regular physical activity thus bolsters overall well-being, ameliorating acid reflux symptoms.

Stress Management and Relaxation Techniques

1. Stress's Impact on Acid Reflux:

The correlation between stress and aggravated acid reflux symptoms is substantial. Stress triggers increased stomach acid production, weakens the lower esophageal sphincter, and induces muscle tension in the digestive system. Thus, integrating stress management and relaxation techniques is integral to holistic acid reflux treatment.

2. Effective Relaxation Practices:

Techniques like deep breathing exercises, meditation, yoga, and progressive muscle relaxation have demonstrated efficacy in stress reduction and alleviating acid reflux symptoms. These practices induce relaxation, mitigate muscle tension, and lower stress hormone production, collectively contributing to acid reflux management.

3. Mindfulness and Cognitive-Behavioral Strategies:

Beyond relaxation techniques, mindfulness practices, cognitive-behavioral therapy, and stress-reducing activities are instrumental in stress management. Incorporating these strategies into daily routines aids in diminishing stress's impact on the digestive system, fostering relief from acid reflux symptoms.

Significance of Quality Sleep

1. Sleep's Impact on Acid Reflux:

Quality sleep forms a cornerstone of holistic acid reflux management. Disrupted sleep patterns, insomnia, and sleep disorders heighten acid reflux symptoms by disrupting the digestive system and elevating stress levels. Prioritizing quality sleep is thus imperative for reducing the severity of acid reflux symptoms.

2. Establishing Healthy Sleep Habits:

Structuring a consistent sleep schedule, cultivating a conducive sleep environment, and practicing good sleep hygiene are pivotal in ensuring quality sleep. Additionally, integrating pre-sleep relaxation techniques like meditation and deep breathing contributes to better sleep quality and symptom alleviation.

3. Weight Management and Sleep Practices:

Maintaining a healthy weight, refraining from large meals before bedtime, and elevating the head of the bed are practices that further enhance sleep quality. These considerations mitigate the likelihood of nocturnal acid reflux incidents, providing comprehensive relief.

By focusing on enhancing the quality of sleep, individuals can effectively manage acid reflux, promoting a more holistic approach to overall well-being.

Chapter 7

Addressing Queries and Navigating Challenges in Acid Reflux Management

Embarking on the journey to manage acid reflux with the aid of an acid reflux cookbook can present various hurdles and inquiries. This chapter aims to alleviate common concerns and provide troubleshooting tips to ensure your progression towards improved health remains steadfast.

Distinguishing Food Intolerances from Acid Reflux Triggers

1. Understanding Food Intolerances:

Food intolerances stem from the body's struggle to digest specific foods, resulting in symptoms like bloating and stomach pain. Although uncomfortable, these symptoms are distinct from acid reflux. Recognizing and discerning your food intolerances is vital for making informed dietary decisions and averting unnecessary discomfort.

2. Identifying Acid Reflux Triggers:

Acid reflux triggers are particular foods or drinks that can worsen acid reflux symptoms. These triggers vary among individuals, with common culprits including spicy foods, citrus fruits, and caffeine. Identifying personal triggers empowers you to make mindful dietary choices, effectively managing acid reflux and mitigating the frequency and severity of symptoms.

3. Troubleshooting Triggers:

Employing a food diary to document your intake and corresponding symptoms proves helpful in troubleshooting potential triggers. This diary offers valuable insights into your personal triggers, facilitating informed decisions about your diet and lifestyle.

Maneuvering Social Situations and Dining Out

1. Navigating Restaurant Menus:

When dining out, perusing the menu beforehand and pinpointing potential acid reflux triggers or alternatives is beneficial. Many restaurants are accommodating and willing to adjust dishes to align with dietary restrictions. Communicating your needs to the server or chef ensures your meal is prepared in harmony with your dietary preferences.

2. Open Communication in Social Settings:

Engaging in open conversations with friends and family about your dietary restrictions and health goals can foster understanding and support. Explaining the impact of acid reflux triggers on your well-being encourages a supportive environment in social settings.

Sustaining Progress and Preventing Relapses

1. Consistency in Diet and Lifestyle:

Maintaining progress in acid reflux management necessitates unwavering consistency in adhering to a reflux-friendly diet and lifestyle. This entails meticulous meal planning, practicing mindful eating, and staying informed about potential triggers and their effects on symptoms.

2. Incorporating Stress Management:

Integrating stress-management techniques and regular physical activity contributes to overall well-being and fortifies efforts in acid reflux management. Stress can exacerbate symptoms, and adopting practices like meditation or yoga aids in stress reduction.

3. Utilizing Symptom Diaries:

Regularly monitoring progress and symptoms through a symptom diary offers valuable insights. This documentation enables you to identify patterns or triggers affecting acid reflux. Regular reviews empower you to proactively address challenges and make necessary adjustments in support of your ongoing health.

By addressing these common concerns and implementing effective strategies, you can navigate challenges in acid reflux management with confidence, fostering a sustained journey towards improved well-being.

Conclusion

The "Acid Reflux Cookbook for Beginners" emerges as an invaluable resource for individuals grappling with acid reflux, offering a transformative guide to enhancing their dietary and lifestyle choices for symptom relief. This cookbook stands out by providing a holistic understanding of acid reflux, delving into its origins, symptoms, and potential complications. It not only imparts practical insights into managing the condition through dietary and lifestyle adjustments but also explores medicinal and alternative treatment avenues.

The recipes within the cookbook are thoughtfully crafted to be gentle on the digestive system, minimizing the risk of triggering acid reflux symptoms. Beyond their palatable nature, these recipes serve as a nutritional compass, enabling individuals with acid reflux to relish a diverse array of foods without exacerbating their condition. The cookbook extends its utility by furnishing valuable tips and guidelines on meal planning, grocery shopping, and navigating dining-out scenarios, empowering individuals to sustain a wholesome and gratifying diet.

A distinguishing feature of the "Acid Reflux Cookbook for Beginners" lies in its unwavering emphasis on whole, natural foods. The recipes showcase an array of fruits, vegetables, whole grains, lean proteins, and healthy fats, all renowned for their digestive health benefits and risk reduction for acid reflux. By prioritizing these nutrient-dense ingredients, the cookbook facilitates the adoption of a balanced and nourishing diet, thereby supporting overall well-being.

Moreover, the cookbook advocates for mindful eating and portion control, fostering a paradigm shift that enables individuals with acid reflux to steer clear of overindulgence and better manage their symptoms. This mindfulness-oriented approach encourages individuals to savor meals, attune to bodily signals, and make discerning choices about their dietary preferences. Particularly advantageous for those with acid reflux, this approach aids in identifying and avoiding trigger foods, curbing overeating tendencies, and mitigating the likelihood of uncomfortable symptoms.

In summation, the "Acid Reflux Cookbook for Beginners" stands as a trove of insightful information and pragmatic counsel for individuals contending with acid reflux. By delivering a repertoire of delectable and nutritious recipes, alongside practical advice for navigating the intricacies of managing acid reflux, the cookbook empowers individuals to assert control over their diet and lifestyle. Whether one is embarking on the initial steps of acid reflux management or navigating the challenges over the years, this cookbook emerges as an indispensable tool for those endeavoring to instill positive changes. With its core tenets rooted in whole, natural foods, mindful eating, and portion control, the "Acid Reflux Cookbook for Beginners" serves as an instrumental guide for individuals to relish delicious, gratifying meals while mitigating symptoms and fortifying their overall health.

Dear Reader, Did you enjoy this book? What are your thoughts? Kindly drop a review to share your impression of this book....... Thanks!